A DOCTOR'S PATH TO HEALING

Dr. Audrey Gilchrist Johnston

Dedication

I dedicate this book to the memory of my beloved late parents Richard and Mary Gilchrist who gave me the best start in life any child could have.

"Train up a child in the way he should go, and when he is old, he will not depart from it" Proverbs 22:6.

A DOCTOR'S PATH TO HEALING

Publisher's statement: Throughout this book the love for our God is such that whenever we refer to Him we honour with capitals. On the other hand, when referring to the devil, we refuse to acknowledge him with any honour to the point of violating grammatical rule and withholding capitalisation.

Published by

Maurice Wylie Media
Your Inspirational & Christian Book Publisher

For more information visit
www.MauriceWylieMedia.com

Contents

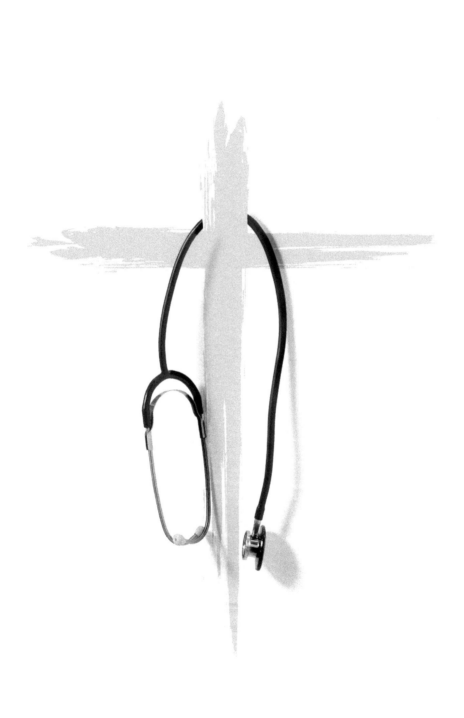

Foreword

I first got to know Audrey Johnston when the multi-church Healing on the Streets (HOTS) team in Ballymena was started back in 2016. Audrey has been a faithful, and faith-filled, member of the team since the start, and has brought to the team both an expertise and a strong faith in God both to save to the utmost and to heal miraculously; the one coming from her medical career as a general practitioner, the other from her remarkable relationship with Jesus and experiences of miraculous healings in her own life.

Faithful and faith-filled are just two qualities in Audrey that will strike the reader in this very readable account of her life thus far. Every page oozes a quiet determination to press through in obedience to the heavenly calling, a preparedness to persevere in her quest to see God at work in her own life, and a courage to endure adversity and at times agonising pain, often with a gritty cheerfulness and humour.

The main focus of this book is the fascinating and challenging account of six significant healings that Audrey has experienced in her own body, at least two of them "incurable" diseases. As she says, each one involved a different journey of simple faith, trust, and obedience, as well as what she describes as a willingness to "push through the crowd" to lay hold of the promise of God.

This is much more than a simple account of some remarkable healings; the story is set in the narrative of her life journey, from her childhood faith, the influence of her parents, and others, to her finding God for herself and proving Him in every aspect of her life.

From start to finish, this autobiography reveals someone with a very personal, intimate and interactive faith in the Living Saviour, from her childhood responses to God, to her call to medicine and then to "Carry My Healing" to others, both at home and overseas. There are lessons here in godly decision-making, guidance, identifying and defeating the lies and deceptions of the enemy, forgiveness of self and others, laying hold of the miraculous, the power of simply believing, and keeping one's healing.

Simplistic this book is not – and there are some great insights and answers to questions such as: should I stay on my meds? What if healing doesn't come? What, if anything, is preventing my healing? And how do I stay healed?

Nor is the book formulaic. What has been Audrey's life secret? Well, I will leave you, the reader, to work that out for yourself. However, there is a chapter towards the end entitled "Why me?" which reveals what has become clear along the way. Yet Audrey would be the first to admit she is not any more special than you or I. On three occasions she uses two simple words that, for me, sum up Audrey's not-so-secret secret: "My Jesus." If her story tells us anything, it is that the key to experiencing the reality of Jesus in one's life is to live that life in a relationship of love, trust and obedience.

Dr Jonathan Leakey, PhD PGCE.

Introduction

I was a medical doctor who could not find healing in medicine. This physician could not heal herself. But Jesus could, and He did. "By His stripes I am healed" became more than a nice Bible verse to me; it became my story on my journey to divine healing. This is the true story of a healing journey with Jesus. I invite you to follow my journey.

I began to have symptoms of ankylosing spondylitis in childhood, which worsened through my teenage years. However, I obeyed God's call to study medicine, and it was during my studies that I self-diagnosed. This was later confirmed by a consultant rheumatologist, and medical treatment was prescribed. I was also diagnosed with multiple sclerosis, which only affected my right arm. At that time, no drug treatment was available.

Due to increasing health issues and work stresses, I took early retirement from my work as a General Practitioner in 2010, but I was still determined to serve God in whatever way I could. After more than two years of seeking God's will for my future, He touched me, and I was miraculously healed from ankylosing spondylitis and called to "Carry My Healing to others." A few weeks later, I was also healed from multiple sclerosis; praise God!

As time passed, other conditions afflicted me, but God has always been faithful to heal me. I have learned so much on this journey about how to receive God's healing and how we so often prevent ourselves from receiving it. I am still learning. By no means do I have all the answers, but if my story helps someone else on their journey to healing, it is not written in vain.

To God be all the glory.

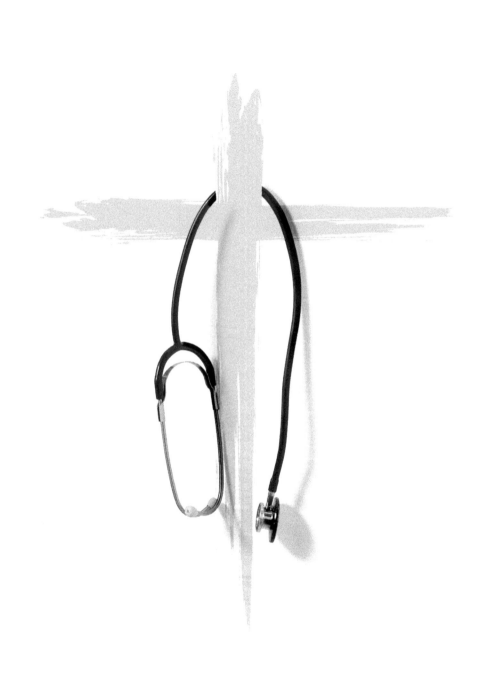

Chapter 1

My Early Years

I grew up on a small farm in the Broughshane area of County Antrim in Northern Ireland, in the townland of Caugherty, to be exact. Broughshane then was just a small country village with basic shops, churches, and the primary school, which I attended. The village existed then to serve the needs of the local farming community and the two woollen mills. It has been transformed over the years and has won many British and international awards for conservation and floral displays.

As a child, I loved the farming way of life and especially loved the beauty of God's creation. I had no fear of animals, and I'm told that as a very young child I used to love to go in to the pig houses and try to straighten out the pigs' curly tails! I was also very fond of our hens, and from a young age, I was very adept at collecting the newly laid eggs. I'm told I was also very brave about putting my hand under a broody hen (or a "clocking hen" in the local dialect) to claim the eggs she wanted to hatch. Such hens were prone to peck an adult's hand, but never mine. The family farm was mixed as was common in the 1960s, so we also had cattle for fattening. My uncles had milking cows, which were of course milked by hand, and learning to milk was a great achievement. That meant we drank unpasteurised milk, which did us no harm and tasted lovely.

Mixed farming also meant growing crops then, mainly potatoes and barley, and cutting hay to provide food for the cattle in winter as well as barley straw for bedding after the grain was harvested. I really was an outdoor girl. My memories of helping in the hay fields would have been during the school summer holidays in July and August. I thought I was some girl when I was strong enough to lift a bale of hay! They were rectangular then, of course, not the round bales wrapped in black plastic one would see nowadays. Planting potatoes (or dropping potatoes, as we called it) would have been done in the spring, yet I remember sitting on the machine and dropping seed potatoes at regular intervals into the prepared drills. Harvesting, or "potato gathering," was in the autumn, so I must have been out in the fields as soon as the homework was done. I wasn't as good at gathering, for it was a job that made most backs ache then, and mine was no exception.

I think my favourite aspect of country life was helping my father in the vegetable and flower garden. The beauty of flowers was something that always amazed me and still does. When I look at a flower, I see the perfection of God's creation. I don't ever remember seeing a flower any other way, and I am thankful for my father's influence in that.

Daddy had a heart condition called rheumatic heart disease, which affected the valves of his heart. This was a consequence of developing rheumatic fever in childhood, a condition never seen today because penicillin given on time for the relevant throat infection prevents that disease. Daddy was born in 1922, and penicillin was only discovered in 1928 and not yet available when he would have needed it. I tell you this because, although Daddy was a farmer, he was not physically able to do the most strenuous types of farm-work, and he and I became very close companions. His brothers did the heavy work on our farm and their own. I know it was my father's Christian influence that taught me to see the wonder and beauty of creation and our Creator, God. But I'll tell you more about Daddy later.

I was blessed to be brought up in a Christian home and go to Sunday school, church, and the Junior Girls' Auxiliary. The motto of the latter organisation was *"I can do all things through Christ who strengthens me,"* Philippians 4:13. How precious that scripture would become to me in later life.

I learned through all these Godly influences that God loved me and that He sent His son Jesus Christ to die for me so that I could be rescued from a life of sin and have the promise of eternal life in Heaven. As a young child, I knew I would need to accept Jesus someday, but maybe not just yet, because very devout Christian people (like my Sunday school teacher) could be a bit peculiar, and I wasn't ready to become peculiar yet! So thought a seven or eight-year-old me. Wasn't God so merciful? Of course, that dear lady was not at all peculiar, as I came to understand. She loved the Lord Jesus Christ so much that He influenced every word she spoke and everything she did. She had no agenda of her own. Her only interest was serving her Lord with all her being. She eventually became a missionary in Zaire, as it was then, now the Democratic Republic of Congo. A few years ago she went to be with Jesus. I suspect that to some people, I may seem as peculiar now as my friend did then, and I pray all such will see beyond that as I did. That change in a person when they become a Christian occurs because 2 Corinthians 5:17 tells us, *"Therefore, if anyone is in Christ, he is a new creation; old things have passed away; behold, all things have become new."* The more a person is obedient to 2 Corinthians 6:17, *"Come out from among them and be separate says the Lord,"* the more Christ-like they become.

I remember receiving a Sunday school prize book called Jungle Doctor, which was to have a lasting impact. It was about a missionary doctor in a Swahili-speaking African country. The innocent nine-year-old thought that missionary work would be such a good thing to do and began memorising the few words of Swahili that that little book contained. Bwana meant Lord or Master. Whoever chose that book for me probably never knew the seeds it would sow, but more about that later.

During my childhood years, I often had joint pains, especially in my knees. In the 1960s, the diagnosis was "growing pains," and the doctor's remedy was to rub olive oil into my joints. My mother observed that it made hair grow on my legs but did little else! Certainly, it made no difference to the knee pains. It was painful to kneel down for any length of time to work in our beloved garden. It was painful if we had to sit cross-legged at school. I couldn't run very well, so I was the last in every race, and I hated PE and games at school. I was the girl nobody wanted in their team, always the last to be chosen. I also started to have backache around the age of eight or nine, and I remember how Daddy used to sit by my bed rubbing my back at night to help ease the discomfort and help me fall asleep.

At the age of eleven and a half, tragedy struck our family. My very much-loved father died of heart failure due to rheumatic heart disease, and my world collapsed around me. This was 1970. Daddy's health had been deteriorating for five months, but nobody thought to warn children that we would soon be parted from him—on Saturday May 23, at 6.50pm to be exact. I did not get to say goodbye to the person I loved most in all the world. I didn't see him in the coffin and didn't get to go to his funeral. It just wasn't the "done thing" then. No one had thought that children might need grief counselling in those days. It was just around the end of the "children should be seen and not heard" era and also the beginning of "The Troubles" in Northern Ireland. Although I loved my mother and younger sister dearly, I had been a "Daddy's girl." I had spent so much time outside with him on the farm and in the garden, while my sister spent more time with our mother. How was I going to live on without my precious Daddy?

On the fiftieth anniversary of Daddy's death, I wrote the following tribute to him and posted it on Facebook:

> *"On this day fifty years ago, May 23, 1970, I had to part with the best human being I have ever known. That person was my father, forever Daddy to me. I was eleven when he died of rheumatic heart disease, having had rheumatic fever in childhood. He was forty-eight. How precious my memories of him have been.*

Daddy was the gentlest, wisest, most caring person in my life. He was a farmer with only an elementary education, yet his understanding of life and people was beyond that of a philosopher. He was no theologian, but he knew and loved God. I remember him explaining to me what communion was about one night when he came home after a Presbyterian pre-communion service. I still remember the smell of his Sunday suit and the faintest hint of Old Spice as I snuggled up to him during the sermon in church. He liked us to listen to the song "Scarlet Ribbons" because it was about a child praying for the impossible in the natural and waking up to find her prayer had been answered. Daddy wanted us to understand the power and importance of prayer.

I have really special memories of us working in the garden together. Every scent of a pansy or a sweet pea takes me back, if only for a moment. Daddy saw the hand of God in His creation and taught me to do the same. Daddy truly cared for the animals he looked after—a man who could herd cattle without using a stick, a man who couldn't bear to drown kittens (as was the practice in those days; no vet bills for spaying).

He wasn't a soft man. It took strength of character to be as gentle and kind as Daddy was. I remember him being so very upset by the Aberfan disaster in 1966. The thought of children dying so tragically, and the grief of their parents moved him to tears. I was between 7 and 8 then and began to share Daddy's compassion. A child at school died of meningitis, and again I saw that same beautiful compassion.

Of course, Daddy's greatest earthly love was for his wife and two little girls. "Keep the wee girls happy," he so often said to Mammy, and she never forgot. I never remember being scolded by him; just gently taught how best to live. That sort of teaching sticks with a child. He taught me humility but at the same time self-respect. "Remember you're as good as anyone else, but never look down on anybody." That was wisdom to a very timid nine-year-old, and something I was to think of often as I grew up. I don't suppose he knew how long he would live, but he must have realised his time would be limited by his heart condition.

Daddy died exactly one week before I received my 11-Plus results. There was no excitement. Nobody had even remembered the results were due that day. Our grief was too profound for it to matter much at first. But life went on. Daddy didn't know I got to Ballymena Academy; he didn't know I went on to university and became a doctor. He didn't know that I married and was blessed with three children, and now grandchildren. He didn't know that in my retirement, I delight in the opportunity to preach the gospel and share the love of God in Kenya. But his good influence in my formative years went with me and, I hope, will continue while I live. How often over the years I asked myself, "What would Daddy do?" "What would Daddy say?" And I do sometimes wonder how different my life might have been if Daddy had lived on, but that's pointless. Parenthood is a huge responsibility. Most of us get some of it right and some of it wrong, but, to me, Daddy got it all correct.

I'm not one of those people who believes our loved ones are watching over us from Heaven. I'm not even certain if we'll recognise each other there because I will spend eternity worshipping my Lord and Saviour. But if I can take my eyes off Jesus for even a moment, I hope I can meet with Daddy again."

So how did I live without my Daddy? In Northern Ireland, we change schools from primary to either secondary or grammar school depending on the result of the exam referred to above. So by September 1970, a quiet little grief-stricken girl from a small primary school had to change schools to the large Ballymena Academy. I had never been good at making friends anyway; I was always an introvert, but this situation was just about as impossible as an eleven-year-old could imagine. There was no counselling or support in schools then. I was expected to just get on with it. Unfortunately, when chatting to new people the subject would turn to family and a common question was "What does your dad do?" at which point I would burst into tears. In French and German conversation classes, I had to quickly discover how to say "My father is dead" in the relevant language. One might have thought that in a class of thirty children, there might have been one other child in the same situation, but no, I was the only grieving fatherless child in the class, so I could find no-one who had any idea of my suffering. The loneliness and heartache were indescribable.

I went through two to three years of questioning all I thought I knew about God. How could a God who loved me take my Daddy from me? I would eventually understand that God took my father home to be with Himself, as his work on earth must have been finished. Reaching that understanding and accepting it took time, which God lovingly and mercifully gave me, and as time passed, I knew that God was awaiting a response from me. I did not know until later that two Christian girls in my class at school had been praying for my salvation.

It was Harvest Sunday 1973, October 7, to be precise. God had been drawing me since the middle of that summer. During the summer, I had prayed and asked Jesus to be my Saviour, confessing my faith in Him, but somehow, I didn't feel any different. I didn't have the peace and joy that I expected to receive, so I suspect that first prayer had not been completely sincere for some reason, and God knew it. I went to church as normal that harvest Sunday. The church was beautifully decorated, as churches in rural areas tend to be for Harvest Sunday. I was captivated by the beauty of God's creation all around me. Nobody but God could have created such beauty and goodness. I don't remember who the preacher was that day; I don't remember the sermon, I don't remember the hymns; but I remember the conviction of the Holy Spirit and knowing I must wait no longer. The God of all creation was calling me to be His. I remember fighting back the tears and telling God I would pray properly when I got home. People didn't burst into tears of repentance in a Presbyterian church back then.

When we got home, I ran upstairs and knelt by my bed and surrendered my life to the Lord Jesus Christ. How I love to remember that moment, the beginning of my journey with Jesus, and the tears I shed. I don't suppose a fourteen-year-old could have committed any serious sins—I've committed worse as a saved adult and repented—but only other born-again believers know the joy and the absolute relief of knowing my sins had been washed away by the cleansing blood of my precious Saviour. Burdens are definitely lifted at Calvary, and only at Calvary. It's so wonderful how God knows exactly how to draw each of us as individuals because He knows us so intimately. He knew He could speak to me through flowers. He knows how to speak to you and your loved ones too.

Throughout my teens, I continued to have the knee and back pains described earlier, but I had a quiet determination not to let health issues beat me. I was a fairly bright student at Ballymena Academy and thought I would rather like to become a science teacher. My back used to ache sitting on the stools in the science laboratories, but I kept that to myself. Around the age of sixteen, God began to speak into my life in various ways, all directing me to a career in medicine.

Chapter 2

The Call to be a Doctor

As I said at the end of the previous chapter, when I was 16 years of age and approaching O-level examinations, I became aware that God was calling me to a career in medicine. That is a time of decision for many young people, and it must be difficult to make such a decision without trusting in God's guidance. I wanted to serve God, but I thought I could serve Him as a teacher. It was uncomfortable to realise that God was saying otherwise!

I still often thought of Daddy and how doctors had done all they could to help him. What would it be like to be able to help people who were ill? A careers teacher speaking of teaching as a career told me, "Those who can, do. Those who cannot, teach" What a strange statement from a teacher, but she wanted me to understand that I fell into the category of those who could! But mainly, the call to medicine came directly from God—that 'knowing' in my spirit that my Heavenly Father was talking to me. How I protested! "I'm not clever enough. I would never get the grades I would need." "I'm far too squeamish; I couldn't do it." To the latter, God always reminded me *"My grace is sufficient for thee."*[1] His strength certainly was perfect in my weakness, as the passage of time showed. Of course, I did achieve the academic standards required by the grace of God alone. And I remembered *"I can do all things through Christ who strengthens me."*[2] So I said yes to my Heavenly Father. I was not going to disobey His clear calling.

[1] 2 Corinthians 12:9.
[2] Philippians 4:13.

I remember thinking one would have to be really healthy to become a doctor, so I suffered a lot in silence. I have no idea where that idea came from! If I needed a medical report to train as a doctor, there would be no mention of the increasingly severe back and knee pain I was suffering. I would do whatever I had to in order to obey God's calling on my life. Wrong thinking, of course! There was to be a lot of wrong but well-intentioned thinking in my life as a young Christian! God was so wonderfully gracious and patient with me. Only my merciful Father God could have tolerated the foolish thinking of a babe in Christ! Why did I not just ask the Lord to take the pain away?

Obeying God's calling was not necessarily easy. My first hurdle was my A-level exams. It came as a great shock and disappointment when the results came out and I was one point too low in my grades. I could get into any other university course as my grades were certainly good, just one point too low for medicine at Queen's University in Belfast. I could study pharmacy or psychology in Belfast, or I could study medicine in Dublin. I felt it would be wrong to be far from my mother, who would be alone on the farm during the week if I were in Belfast, and I could not come home every weekend from Dublin. It was such a dilemma for an eighteen-year-old to have to make a decision about. "What am I to do, Lord?" I could not ignore His calling, although I could not understand how I found myself in this predicament. I recall being taken to Belfast by my uncle and aunt, who were both teachers, to meet the Dean of the Faculty of Medicine at Queen's University. I was terrified! As far as I recall, it was at this point that the suggestion of repeating A-level physics and biology was put to me. I already had a grade A in chemistry; I just needed to improve my grade in one of these subjects. That would mean returning to school for an extra year, joining those who had been in the year below me. At that age, a year felt like a long time as well as being somewhat humiliating. However, I decided that was the right option, and at the end of that year, I had the A-level grades I needed to study medicine in Belfast. I began my studies in 1978, just a year later than I originally expected to, and maybe a bit of humiliation was character-building!

Leaving home in the country to live in Belfast during "the troubles" was quite a challenge. For the first year and a half we had lectures in the Medical Biology Centre on the Lisburn Road, so there was little travelling involved. But after that, we were sent on placements to hospitals, and it became necessary, with the help of aunts and uncles and my savings from a summer job, to buy my first car, a blue Mini Clubman. Travelling to the Royal Victoria Hospital regularly meant passing police and army patrols, which we knew were often in the sights of terrorist snipers. I was rarely frightened because I trusted God to keep me safe while I did what He called me to do.

Medical studies are far from easy. I quickly understood why students needed to prove their academic ability with good A-level grades. I have to admit that I did not enjoy the early stages. We studied anatomy, physiology, and biochemistry. I expected to enjoy the latter two, but nothing was as I expected, and it was all quite a struggle. Certain topics were as interesting to me as watching paint dry! Yet I persevered. When we started to study clinical subjects and at last had contact with real patients, everything changed, and I enjoyed every specialty and every attachment. When I was learning how to talk to patients, examine them, and come to a diagnosis, I knew I was walking in God's calling, and I was thankful that I did not give up at the early hurdles.

I remember as a third-year medical student learning about a condition called Ankylosing Spondylitis, often associated with sero-negative arthropathy (inflammation in the joints that is not due to rheumatoid arthritis), and realising that this was my diagnosis. I understand the modern name for the condition is Axial Spondylo-arthropathy. My symptoms were exactly as described in the textbooks. I had pain and stiffness in my spine and difficulty keeping from developing a stooped posture. I was reminded of the woman in Luke 13:10-12: *"Now He was teaching in one of the synagogues on the Sabbath. And behold, there was a woman who had a spirit of infirmity eighteen years, and was bent over and could in no way raise herself up. But when Jesus saw her, He called her to Him and said to her, "Woman, you are loosed from your infirmity.'"* So, I knew that Jesus could heal this condition.

I discovered that in the natural, there was no real cure for this auto-immune condition (which means that one's own immune system attacks various organs, in my case my spine and other joints). There were just drugs to try to reduce the pain and inflammation. And these drugs had side effects. How was I going to work as the symptoms became worse? I would keep it to myself as long as possible in case the diagnosis affected my career prospects. There I was again, as if trying to help God achieve what He had planned for my life! I cringe when I recall such immature thinking and thank God for His mercy and grace. I do hope some readers can relate to the foolish thinking of immature Christians and find encouragement in this book.

I remember increasing back and knee pain during the long ward rounds we did with the consultants who taught us. Anyone who has been an inpatient in a teaching hospital has seen what the medical students go through! But I loved it; it was my calling, and I would battle on. Naturally, the enemy was not impressed by my obedience to my calling, and a further unexpected obstacle was to come.

I graduated as a doctor and took up a post in the Waveney Hospital in Ballymena on August 1, 1983. By mid-September, suddenly, and without any prior symptoms, I was an inpatient in the Royal Victoria Hospital in Belfast with a paralysed right arm and a diagnosis of probable Multiple Sclerosis. I had been working one night in the medical ward when my right arm suddenly became weak and numb, and I had to call a senior colleague to take over from me. I was initially admitted to the Waveney Hospital and subsequently transferred to the Royal Victoria Hospital for further investigation.

Multiple sclerosis is a disease where certain nerves in the spine or particular parts of the brain stop functioning properly. I knew patients with it, some of whom had been bedbound for years. There were no CT scans or MRI scans in 1983 and no drug treatments. The diagnosis was made largely by ruling out other possible causes for my symptoms, what the medical profession calls the differential diagnoses. I had to have a cervical myelogram, which is x-rays taken after the injection of a radio-opaque substance into the fluid surrounding the lumbar spine. The most unpleasant part of the procedure was being strapped into a cradle and rotated so that my head was towards the ground. This allowed the radio-opaque substance to flow by gravity to my neck and show if there was a prolapsed disc, a tumour, or similar problems. The x-rays showed no abnormality, but that was not actually good news for me. That fact, in conjunction with a slight abnormality of the constituents in the fluid around my spine, meant that my diagnosis was probable multiple sclerosis.

Any other possibilities had been ruled out.

During the procedure, I developed a horrendous headache, followed by vomiting if I moved at all. I did not see any improvement in my condition as the days went by, and I thought it pointless to remain any longer in the hospital. I remember suggesting signing myself out of the hospital against medical advice because I was so frustrated, so the doctors agreed to let me go. I knew that my dear mother's unqualified but loving nursing care would help if anything could. We were still in "the Troubles" then, and as my fiancé drove and my mother looked after me, I remember the car being hit by a brick as we drove under a flyover. We could all have been killed, but God was watching over us.

So that was where medicine was in 1983, and the treatment plan was to wait and see. I was on sick leave from work and definitely did not want colleagues or superiors to know the presumed diagnosis. I gradually regained movement in my arm and hand but was left with persistent numbness and a lack of awareness of position sense (proprioception), which meant I had to look at my hand and fingers to use them effectively. I finally had to confess to the consultant I was working under and was allowed to return to work. It was difficult to adapt, yet somehow, with great determination and despite being right-handed, I found a way to use my hand for all I needed to do at work, including delivering babies and performing surgical procedures. The patients never knew, and my work colleagues noticed nothing because God's strength was perfect in my weakness.

My husband and I married on October 8, just a few weeks after my diagnosis of MS. Despite my health problems, we were blessed with three very much-loved children.

Childbirth was complicated due to the increasing deformity and stiffness in my back and pelvis, but my precious babies were worth all the difficulties. In my third labour under epidural, I remember the anaesthetist saying that he hoped this was my last baby, as he didn't think a needle could be inserted into my spine again. Wise advice indeed, and a healthy daughter and two healthy sons were more than enough blessings for us.

Family life and work life were busy. My husband and I had met in the summer between school and university at a Christian event. He was such a great support through all the difficulties of student life and my health problems. However, he felt no call to missionary work, and somehow memories of Jungle Doctor were buried. I wasn't medically fit to work abroad anyway, or so I told myself.

It was in August 1989 that I had such a severe flare-up of joint problems that I was admitted to the hospital, and investigations confirmed what I had known for several years, namely that I had Ankylosing Spondylitis, associated with the tissue type HLAb27. From then on, I was prescribed all sorts of medications and had numerous steroid injections into several joints. By this stage, I was a general practitioner and accepted that the village in which I worked was my mission field. I cannot break confidentiality, but God did use me in those days, and there are people serving Him today for whom I prayed. There are also people with the Lord today for whom I had prayed. I truly believed with all my heart that God could heal, and I prayed for patients, with or without their knowledge. Sometimes I didn't know what was wrong with a patient, and God would lead me to the diagnosis. Throughout all my working years, I suffered agonising pain. Sometimes I wept with pain on the way to work but stood on the promise that *"They that wait upon the Lord shall renew their strength. They shall mount up with wings as eagles. They shall run and not grow weary and shall walk and not faint."* Isaiah 40:31. By the time I reached the Health Centre,

I had strength for another day. "One day at a time, sweet Jesus," the words of a popular gospel song at that time.

There had been a lot of paramilitary activity in the village prior to my arrival, and I had some of the aftermath to deal with. Then the drug problem arrived in the form of heroin, and rumours went around among drug users about this certain lady GP who was not judgmental and really tried to help. Some said I had made a rod for my own back, but when I meet people now who were once addicts and are now happily employed family men and women, I am glad I sometimes went the extra mile. I don't know why I had a special compassion for addicts, as it's a problem I've only ever encountered professionally. But God knows.

Back to my journey now. My wrong thinking for most of my adult life was that there was a purpose for my suffering in that I was a more compassionate doctor because of my own experience of pain. So, was I a better doctor than all my healthy colleagues? I was better than some and not as good as others, but my suffering had nothing to do with it. Nothing but the indwelling presence of the Holy Spirit influenced how good a doctor I was. We read in Galatians 5:22-23 that the fruit of the Spirit is love, joy, peace, long-suffering, kindness, goodness, faithfulness, gentleness, and self-control. So, if I was a bit more caring, sweet-natured, patient, kind, and tolerant than I otherwise might have been, it was nothing at all to do with my own personal suffering, but the work of the Holy Spirit.

When the enemy tells a Christian a lie, he is cunning enough to make it plausible. Just as a money forger doesn't make £9 notes, the enemy knows how to make his lies believable. He is, after all, the father of all lies.[3] I loved my Lord with all my being, yet the enemy deceived me. What baffled me was that I had loved and served my precious Lord for decades, and yet the enemy still deceived me. Jesus said, *"My sheep hear my voice."* John 10:27. I did hear my Lord's voice so often. After all, everyone who is born again has heard the voice of God in conviction, or they wouldn't have been saved. And I so often depended on hearing my Lord's guidance with difficult medical problems and for guidance in

---

[3]John 8:44.

other areas of my life. So how did the enemy succeed in deceiving me with that idea? Maybe all I needed was someone to tell me I was wrong.

Chapter 3

Healing of Ankylosing Spondylitis

After twenty years of excellent care by the same consultant rheumatologist for whom I have nothing but praise and respect, by the time I was 50, he advised that both of my hip joints were so worn that joint replacements were my only option. Something made me say "No". Two hip replacements were something I did not feel ready to face. Walking had become extremely painful, and I was exhausted with pain and stressful administrative situations in work. When I was 40, I felt that God was telling me, or maybe giving me permission, to retire at the age of 50. I was actually 51 when I finally retired with a full pension on health grounds.

My body had become so frail, but my mind was still sharp and active, and my desire was still to serve my Lord and Saviour somehow. So, what was I to do with the rest of my life? Looking back, I must have spent about two and a half years seeking God's will for my life and fervently desiring to find another way to serve Him.

One Sunday in June 2012, my daughter invited me to go to a Pentecostal church with her. I had heard good reports about the church, but I loved the church I had attended since childhood. It was appropriate, however, for me to change churches, as I had been Spirit-filled sometime in the 1990s, just through praying and asking Jesus to give me whatever gifts He wanted me to have. Wow! What an experience!

One Sunday in autumn 2012, I was in such severe pain that I was using two walking sticks and had difficulty standing up to worship, despite taking the maximum dose of tramadol, an anti-inflammatory tablet called indomethacin, and a disease-modifying anti-rheumatic drug (DMARD) called sulphasalazine. At the end of the service, the Pastor (who has asked to not be named so that all the glory will go to God) came to me and asked about my health condition. That was the first time we had spoken, and I was touched by his obvious concern. I told him about ankylosing spondylitis and being told I needed two hip replacements, and I also shared my foolish belief about my suffering having made me a more compassionate doctor. I hadn't thought to question why I was still suffering but retired. The Pastor advised me that I was believing a lie from the enemy and that I should go home and pray about it. He did not offer to pray for me; rather, this was something I needed to do myself.

That is exactly what I did. I lay on my bed that Sunday afternoon and poured out my heart to my heavenly Father. I asked Him to forgive me for my wrong belief and to teach me His truth about His desire to heal. I felt such a burden being lifted off me as I repented for believing that God had used sickness in my life. I asked God what I needed to do to be healed and received a clear answer: *"You do not have because you do not ask"*, James 4:2. How simple yet profound! I had always known that God could heal. I had prayed for others, but I had never once asked God to heal me! I just assumed if He wanted to heal me, He would. So, I lay on my bed and asked God to heal me, to take away all the pain and inflammation in my joints, and He did exactly that. I went to church that evening with no walking sticks, knowing God had done something so amazing I could hardly take it in at first. God was so merciful to me for I have to admit it took me a couple of weeks to realise that I was completely and totally healed from ankylosing spondylitis, and as I write this over 10 years later, I remain completely and totally healed because of what Jesus did… *"But He was wounded for our transgressions, He was bruised for our iniquities; The chastisement for our peace was upon Him, And by His stripes we are healed."* Isaiah 53:5. How I thank the Lord for what He suffered so that I could be healed. At one point, when I was praying and worshipping God for the miracle I had received, God spoke to me, saying "Now carry My healing to others." That was my call to a healing ministry.

Obviously, as I was now pain-free, it seemed logical to stop all medication to relieve pain. I had been on the maximum recommended dose of the opiate analgesic tramadol for many years. It had never occurred to me that I could have become addicted to prescribed medication. I certainly had no psychological withdrawal symptoms or cravings whatsoever. But a few days after stopping taking tramadol, I had to accept the uncomfortable fact that I was physically addicted to this drug. I was sweating and trembling like a heroin addict needing the next fix! So here was my reason for always having a particular sympathy for addicts; God knew what was ahead of me! I decided my best plan would be to wean off tramadol gradually. I would endure some physical symptoms but would still be able to function. If I remember rightly, I reduced my daily dose by 50mg once a week. Finally, I was down to 50mg daily, and I hoped after all these weeks that stopping would be easy. That was not the case. I took my last tramadol 50mg on December 25, 2012, and advised the family that thereafter Mum would go cold turkey! I did indeed spend a few days in bed sweating and shivering, but by the New Year I was fine. I assume that no matter what strong analgesia I had been taking, I would have gone through the same experience. Tramadol is maybe less addictive than some other medication I could have taken. My symptoms were unpleasant for a few weeks but worth enduring to be drug-free at last. Of course, if I hadn't wanted to stop my medication, I probably didn't have to, but I wanted to because my Lord and Saviour had healed me and I needed nothing but Him.

A few weeks after my healing, I was baptised by total immersion, something I had desired since being born again in 1973. Second only to being born again, that is my most precious memory. All the other people being baptised that night had been saved a few weeks or months previously. I was saved 39 years at the time. The joy of obeying God's Word and being baptised as Jesus was is indescribable.

My only complaint was that it was too quick, yet I remember it as if in slow motion. The lukewarm water came up around my cheeks, and I can only liken it to being hugged by Jesus Himself. My past was completely left behind in the water, and I arose as a new creation.

May I suggest that if the church you attend only offers sprinkling of babies, I have since learned that many churches who practise full water baptism are willing to baptise non-members provided they are born-again Christians without the expectation of subsequently joining their church. I had wanted all those years to be baptised in order to obey the scriptures, but I had no idea what church to approach about it. I was later told by a friend from another denomination that he could have arranged my baptism years ago but didn't think to offer as he assumed I had been baptised when I was saved.

By no means am I trying to encourage anyone to leave a church where they are happy, have good fellowship, and receive good teaching. It's just that water baptism is a tremendous blessing to miss out on and could even be a step further towards your healing. So, swallow your pride and ask a church that does perform water baptism if you can be baptised. You certainly will not regret it.

Chapter 4

Multiple healings follow

Healing of Multiple Sclerosis

This is by no means the end of my journey to complete healing. Although now pain-free, I still had a numb right arm due to Multiple Sclerosis.

Having experienced God's healing touch on my spine, hips, and other joints, I wanted my arm and hand healed too and had no doubt that God was able. However, I asked as God had told me, and healing did not come; so, there was another lesson to be learned on this journey.

It was January 2013, and our church had three weeks of prayer and fasting to begin the New Year. I was determined to seek God during that time and find out what I needed to do to receive further healing. Over a period of time, God had taken me back in my memory to the onset of the MS symptoms and showed me something in my life that I had not fully repented of. God had tried to warn me about something, and I did not heed His warning. As I repented of this, I sensed God's promise that He would heal me. I cannot share the full detail of God's warning as it was rather personal, but the detail is not relevant. The important issue is that God reminded me of circumstances around the time of my diagnosis to direct me to repentance. Perhaps someone reading this needs to go on a journey with the Lord and find out if there is a long-forgotten, unconfessed sin.

I remember going to a healing service in church on a Wednesday night, believing I would be healed but thinking someone would have to pray for me. I was sitting with my daughter waiting to go for prayer when, all of a sudden, the numbness left my right hand and arm. I had received my healing! I reached out and touched my daughter's face for the first time with my right hand as tears of joy rolled down my cheeks. As babies, I could not feel my children's soft skin with my right hand, only my left. Now I just wanted to keep touching them! Praise the Lord yet again!

Ten years later, I carry a little reminder that only my family and I know about, and now everyone is going to want a sneaky look at my right forearm! Despite being right-handed and doing relatively strenuous work for a woman, my right forearm is visibly thinner than my left. We have measured it, and there is still a 2cm difference in circumference ten years later. I look at my thinner but completely functional right forearm, and I praise my Lord, by whose stripes I am healed.[4] I thank the Holy Spirit for leading me to the repentance that led to my healing.

In July 2022, I can add a little extra confirmation to this healing, not that it was needed. After the final healing I will write about in this book, doctors thought I might have suffered a mini-stroke and should have an MRI scan of my brain. I didn't agree with them, but I had the procedure anyway. Praise God, the result was perfectly normal. I knew I had not had a stroke, just a bad migraine. However, I thought there might be some scar tissue where the multiple sclerosis had been healed, and praise God, there was no sign of it at all. God had restored all my brain tissue to normal in January 2013!

Healing of Irritable Bowel Syndrome…

I had one other condition that I have not previously mentioned, namely irritable bowel syndrome. I will not go into details, just suffice it to say the symptoms were bad! Any more detail than that would be 'too much information,' as my family would say!

---

[4] 1 Peter 2:24.

Many people prayed for my healing, and I prayed and prayed for myself. Sometimes when I was close to fainting with abdominal pain, all I could do was cry out to the Lord and think of what He suffered for me. I had been able to suffer severe joint pain more easily than severe bowel cramps. I experienced frequent episodes of symptoms from around 1990 until August 2020. In fact, sometimes doctors suspected I had Crohn's disease, but internal examinations and biopsies showed that I did not.

Finally, after 30 years, God led me to understand the root of my problem. For many people who have irritable bowel syndrome, their trigger is stress. Despite my other health issues, a demanding job, and raising a family, I did not feel that I suffered from stress. I was blessed with the peace that passes all understanding,[5] so it puzzled me greatly that I suffered from a disorder usually caused by stress.

During a particularly severe episode, I was pleading that the Lord would heal me or show me what I needed to do to be healed. Suddenly I received a revelation: I was not forgiving myself for past sins that God had already forgiven me for. Somehow my past sins felt still anchored to me, yet scripture teaches, *"Come now, and let us reason together," Says the* Lord, *"Though your sins are like scarlet, They shall be as white as snow; Though they are red like crimson, They shall be as wool"* Isaiah 1:18.

The price had been paid in full by the Lord Jesus Christ, yet when certain forgiven sins would come to mind, I would be overcome by regret and be unforgiving towards myself. I was judging myself when God has declared me righteous in, *"I, even I, am He who blots out your transgressions for My own sake; And I will not remember your sins,"* Isaiah 43:25.

And, *"As far as the east is from the west, So far has He removed our transgressions from us"* Psalm 103:12.

That was a life-changing revelation for me, and I pray it will be for

---

[5] Philippians 4:7.

someone reading this also. I suppose all born-again Christians live with some regrets about past sins and many have to live with their consequences too. However, once our sins are under the blood of Jesus, God remembers them no more. It is the accuser of the brethren, satan, who tries to remind us of our forgiven sins and keep us in bondage to unforgiveness. I now find it helpful to ask God to erase troubling thoughts from my memory and help me to take every thought captive— *"bringing every thought in to captivity to the obedience of Christ"* 2 Corinthians 10:5.

Forgiving ourselves is not helped by the fact that sometimes even other Christians will not forgive us. What right do any of us have to pass judgement on a brother or sister in Christ, about a sin that they have confessed and received God's forgiveness for?

I made an error of judgment in 2009—nothing work-related or illegal, I hasten to add, but a personal matter. I repented shortly after and was most gloriously forgiven and washed afresh in the cleansing blood of Jesus. I wasn't backslidden at the time. I was as close to my Lord as ever. I had known for a long time that the harder life becomes, the more tightly I should cling to my Saviour. To be honest, I was menopausal after surgical removal of my ovaries, and I was mentally quite depressed for a few months, such that I made a decision that otherwise I would not have made. My ovaries were removed because medical advice was that I was at high risk of developing ovarian cancer. In hindsight, I would have been wiser to refuse the surgery and trust God. I really learned from that mistake. However, I am so glad to see the increased publicity about menopausal women needing and deserving support at a difficult time in their lives. It definitely greatly disturbed my thought processes for a while.

My point is that since God declares someone righteous through the sacrifice of the Lord Jesus, what possible right could you or I have to say otherwise?

"Forgive us our trespasses as we forgive those who trespass against us." [6]
Have those words become so familiar that we miss their meaning? I

---

[6] Matthew 6:12.

say the Lord's Prayer every night, just as I have since childhood, but I earnestly try to concentrate on every word, every phrase, to use it as a template for deeper intercession.

Therefore, if I am unforgiving towards someone else, am I happy for God to be unforgiving towards me? Most certainly not! I find that a very sobering thought. I believe in keeping short accounts with God. I repent of my sins as soon as I am convicted, and I most especially pray for the grace to harbour no unforgiveness.

Nelson Mandela said, "Resentment (rooted in unforgiveness) is like drinking poison and then hoping it will kill your enemies." How absolutely true! If I harbour bitterness or resentment rooted in unforgiveness towards someone, they possibly neither know nor care, yet I would be eaten up inside. The longer we hold on to offence, the more toxic it can become and the more it can warp our thought processes, our words, and our relationships with others. We know in the natural that if we keep even good food too long until it spoils, it will eventually become harmful and indeed poisonous. This is even more true of a sin such as unforgiveness. Equally, allowing regret about our past sins to fester in our minds despite knowing God's forgiveness, can have the same outcome and, in my case, led to much physical suffering.

I urge you; if you need to forgive someone, do it now, especially if that someone is yourself.

So that is how I came to receive my healing from irritable bowel syndrome. I know it is a common condition. I pray that someone else will be blessed by my story.

I know it is not God's will for any of His blood-washed children to be tormented by regrets. Jesus came that we might have life and have it more abundantly. A mind tortured by shame, guilt, and regret is not enjoying the abundant life the Lord died to bless us with. I thank God for that deep revelation of His truth and for the healing it brought to me.

Healed of Malaria…

In chapter one, I mentioned reading a children's book called Jungle Doctor and memorising a few words in the Swahili language. Throughout adulthood and up until my healing in 2012, I would not have been physically fit to travel to Africa, and my childhood desire to be a missionary was almost forgotten. But God did not forget!

Just after being healed from ankylosing spondylitis, I got to know a gentleman called Wesley Kerr, who is the founder of Life-line Ministries (Ireland). This ministry works in Kenya, a Swahili-speaking country in East Africa. I got to know Wesley and hear about the work in Kenya while serving alongside him in the senior citizen's ministry in church. I so enjoyed hearing what God was doing in Kenya and offered to help with fundraising for the next mission trip.

It was at a fundraising event in January 2013 that I received confirmation that God was calling me to do more than raise funds! I had confided in my daughter that I did wonder if maybe I could and should go to Kenya, so before going to the fundraising event we prayed that God would give me 'a word' if a mission trip was indeed His will. Wesley was showing photographs of children eating ugali, the staple food in Kenya. Ugali was one of the words in Jungle Doctor that only the Holy Spirit could bring to my remembrance. Suddenly, through that one word from a book read around 1967, God was telling me to go to Kenya in 2013! I remember my daughter wondering how Mum knew any Swahili words! I no longer had any excuse to keep me from going, and I did not want an excuse anyway! God had renewed His call, and I obeyed with delight.

The excitement and anticipation were indescribable, and I got to Kenya for the first time in August 2013. I suspected before going that this would not be my only mission trip, and how right I was. On arriving, something felt familiar, as if I had seen the countryside and villages in my dreams. I instantly loved the people, and it was such a joy to share the word of God and see people saved, healed, and delivered. I had loved working as a doctor, but the fulfilment in ministering to these precious people was on a new level for me. I had truly walked into my calling at last. I had to receive my healing first, and I had to be retired to have time to go. I had also accepted God's call to "carry My healing to others." Only my Creator and heavenly Father could have planned my life like this. To God be the glory!

My message to people working in children's ministry is that you do not know what seeds you are sowing in young lives. My message to people who are seeking God's will for their lives is to persevere. God's timing is not our timing. Why did I not get to Kenya until the age of 54? Only God knows, and what a journey it has been.

At the time of writing in 2023, I have now been to Kenya ten times, the last being in April. Three times I went with mission teams, and seven times I have travelled there "alone" but not alone, as the Lord will never leave me nor forsake me.

As far as I remember, it was in 2017 that I contracted malaria in Kenya. It was entirely my own fault because I had not started to take the preventative medication as early as recommended due to being busy right up until I set off. Mosquitos seem to quite like me, and the first few nibbles infected me. At first, I thought I had meningitis as I had a severe headache, a high temperature and a painful stiff neck. I, of course, had never seen a patient with malaria in Northern Ireland! However, my hosts with no medical qualifications were able to tell me that I had malaria as the symptoms were easily recognisable to them. I do not remember any mention of seeing a doctor or going to hospital. I was probably too ill to move, and my dear friends knew that I had such faith for God's healing. Instead, the Life-line pastors in all of our churches were informed of my condition and began to pray for me. Although delirious with fever, I can clearly remember my dear Kenyan sister in Christ, Pastor Caren, kneeling by the bed and weeping as she prayed for my recovery. I was so delirious I was worrying about the inconvenience for my family arranging the repatriation of my body! So, I needed others to be praying, as I was past being able to pray for myself. By the following day, my symptoms had subsided, and after one further day of rest, I was back out preaching and teaching the Word of God. How amazing is my heavenly Father!

I learned two lessons from this episode. Firstly, and simply, take medication as and when prescribed! My body is the temple of the Lord so I must remember my duties as caretaker and not be careless. Secondly, if unwell, ask others to pray. I became too ill to pray for myself, and I am forever grateful to those who stood in the gap.

Healed of a Torn Supraspinatus Tendon…

It was early in 2020 that I started to notice an odd discomfort in my right collar bone. In due course, I realised it was more uncomfortable when I was knitting, so I stopped knitting. I was working several days every week in the Life-line Ministries charity shop in Ballymena, which we had opened in September 2014, and I had been manager from the beginning.

2020 was the year the coronavirus pandemic struck, and all non-essential retail businesses had to close from mid-March due to the government's attempts to curtail the spread of the infection. I mention this because I thought that this would give me the opportunity to rest my shoulder, and hopefully whatever was wrong would settle. I was, of course, praying that God would heal whatever was causing the discomfort and was determined to persist in prayer until I received healing again. Naturally, with each healing that I received, my faith increased dramatically. What God has done before, He can do again.

Several weeks of relative rest did not help at all. The discomfort progressed to pain, and involved the top and back of my shoulder, and was very much worse when I lay down at night. Friends had prayed for me but still the pain increased.

By November, I was becoming exhausted as the pain was significantly disturbing my sleep, so I decided to speak to my general practitioner about it, and an x-ray was arranged. This showed an abnormality, so

I was referred for an ultrasound scan of my shoulder and, I hoped, a steroid injection to disperse the presumed inflammation.

I had to wait until January 25, 2021, for the ultrasound scan, by which stage I was in absolute agony despite resting in a second lockdown. The doctor who performed the scan was a lovely young man and clearly meticulous in his work. The scan seemed to take such a long time, and I remember terrible pain as I had to move my arm in to various positions to allow clear views of different areas of my shoulder joint. Finally, the doctor began to explain his findings and said that a steroid injection would not be appropriate. I had somehow torn the supraspinatus tendon away from the bone to which it should be attached, and the crucial question was whether it would be possible to repair it surgically. There was other damage and inflammation in my shoulder joint as well, with fluid seeping down around the biceps muscle, which was causing pain down my arm. The doctor was puzzled that I had sustained such an injury without having had an accident of some sort. I had probably done some more strenuous work moving furniture in the charity shop than was wise at my age, but I honestly never experienced any sudden pain when lifting, etc. Anyhow, the next plan was to have an MRI scan to help clarify if surgery would be possible, but I was going to need to see an orthopaedic surgeon, and waiting times had become extremely long—literally years for surgery on the NHS.

Each day, the pain was worse than the day before. I could no longer use my right arm for anything, and I was in the depths of despair and utter physical and mental exhaustion. I decided to see a consultant orthopaedic surgeon privately to at least find out if anything could be done in the natural. I was told that very complex surgery would be required at a cost of £6,000 ($7,500), followed by months of rehabilitation. The surgery should ideally be done as soon as possible, as the supraspinatus muscle was contracting more daily, making the proposed procedure progressively more difficult. I made polite excuses and left to supposedly "think it over."

Jesus paid for my healing on the cross and only asked for my repentance, faith, and surrender. I did not have £6,000, but if I had, I could not justify spending it on me when precious people in Kenya and many other third-world countries live on the verge of starvation. My mind was made up; there would be no private surgery. This was another job for the Lord Jesus Christ, the Great Physician, the Great Surgeon, and Him alone. He had graciously healed me so many times before, so I did not doubt His faithfulness to heal again.

The scripture God gave me for this season was Job 23:10, *"He knows the way that I take; when He has tested me I shall come forth as gold"*. This was going to be a serious test, but what a promise!

This experience was different from all others before it. This was unrelenting agony. If I did fall asleep for a few minutes, I often woke up screaming in pain. Doctors sometimes ask how a patient would describe their pain on a scale of 0 to 10. This was 15 out of 10, completely off the scale! And my Jesus knew it. This was pain I could not bear alone but managed to bear because the Lord, as promised, will never leave me nor forsake me.

I remember reading or hearing at some point that one of the many agonies of crucifixion was dislocation of the shoulder joints due to the weight of the body pulling down on the arms. So my Jesus suffered far worse for me, and when I screamed in agony, He understood. I was so close to my Lord in that agony that I can truly say it was worth it. I was so close to the Lord that I was hearing His voice with beautiful clarity. However, on one occasion, He spoke and really shocked me. I clearly heard "There is not much of Audrey left." What does that mean, Lord? I asked. The answer was Galatians 2:20, *"I have been crucified with Christ; it is no longer I who live but Christ lives in me and the life which I now live in the flesh I live by faith in the Son of God, who loved me and gave Himself for me."* I did not feel that I was being reprimanded. In fact, I sensed the pleasure of the Father. But I was not satisfied, and months of prayer followed, seeking to discover what little bit of the old Audrey was still there. It was definitely challenging, and my healing had nothing to do with that part of my journey. I simply had continued to pray for something that was not God's will and therefore stopped.

As you will already be guessing, the Lord did heal me yet again. Washing and dressing were big problems requiring my husband's help. Getting fully dressed, rather than putting on a clean nightdress, was quite an ordeal reserved for special occasions, of which there were few in lockdown. I did, of course, like to get to church at least on Sundays, even though I was trussed up in a special sling which held my arm close to my body, thus preventing any shoulder movement in any direction. So there I was on May 15, 2021, in church with no awareness of the date, praising God as best I could with my left hand raised. But I don't like lopsided worship! Suddenly, I knew that God was telling me to get the sling off and worship properly. "But Lord," I said, "the tendon that lifts my arm isn't attached!" Isn't God so merciful when He has so little to work on? I have, however, by now learned to do as God says, whether I understand or not. So, off came the sling and praise the Lord, my arm shot up without any pain. Tears of gratitude poured down my cheeks. I had "come forth as gold." I have had no pain or restriction of movement in that shoulder since, and as a Christian physiotherapist has confirmed, it had to be a miracle.

Nobody really can explain why that particular tendon tore. I'm not talking about something like thread or string. The scan reports say it is 17mm wide. A tendon is what we might call a sinew in a piece of beef. That would be some size of a sinew, and I'm not a big person. I was 5'1" all my adult life until the ankylosing spondylitis was healed, and my spine straightened out to its full length, and now I'm 5'2." I was never sporty in my youth due to joint problems but I was reasonably strong for my build. However how could I have torn a tendon three-quarters of an inch thick right off the bone at the top of my shoulder and not know when I did it?

I can only come to one conclusion. I have always loved to worship with my hands raised in praise. Not just a little bit, but both hands raised to the heavens as far as I could reach. Psalm 134:2 says, *"Lift up your hands in the sanctuary and bless the Lord"*. In Hebrew worship, Yadah means lifting the hands and worshipping God in full surrender. I suspect the enemy didn't like to see me doing that and thought he could stop me. No way! As the Bible tells us, *"Greater is He that is in me that he that is in the world,"* 1 John 4:4. To God be the glory yet again. In the mighty name of Jesus, I will worship Him to my last breath!

I have since noted the significance of receiving my healing on May 15, 2021. 15 is simply 5x3. Add the numbers 2021 together, and they come to 5. And May is the fifth month. I see a total of five fives in the date, and five in biblical numerology is the number of grace, goodness, and God's favour towards mankind! Twenty-five symbolises grace upon grace or grace multiplied. What an abundance of God's grace I received that day! It was not until sometime afterwards that I realised the significance of the date on which my Lord chose to heal me. How amazing and glorious are His plans! What a blessing and a privilege to "come forth as gold".

Healed of Angina…

I really did think that the healing of my shoulder would be the last story to relate in this book, but the passage of time has proved otherwise. I don't know if the healing I am about to tell you about now will be my last or not, but this has been a long story that I trust will benefit some readers, and I feel I have delayed publication long enough.

Sometime in 2016 or 2017, I started to get occasional pains in my chest. As time went on, they became a bit worse, sometimes radiating down my arms or through to my back. I suspected angina and confided in one of my most excellent GPs. I had an ECG (heart tracing) done in the health centre, and it was not quite normal but not showing anything alarming. I was referred for a coronary angiogram, a scan which looks in detail at the coronary arteries within the heart muscle. It showed one patch of slight narrowing in the left anterior descending coronary artery, the largest artery going down the front wall of the heart. The cardiologist's advice was to lower my cholesterol as much as possible through diet and medication and see how things would go. I didn't have high blood pressure, wasn't a smoker or drinker, and hadn't a family history of ischaemic heart disease. I was just a bit overweight. That was my only risk factor, as medical people talk about. So, I started to take the statin tablets and ate as healthily as possible. The next blood test showed a good improvement, and all seemed well—except I still had occasional chest pain.

There were no dramatic changes until late 2021 or early 2022. I began to notice that the chest pain was becoming more frequent and severe and occurring with less exertion. I consulted my GP in February 2022 and was prescribed an anti-anginal tablet, which made a great difference. I was also referred for an urgent cardiology assessment, and the opinion was that worsening symptoms despite good cholesterol levels suggested I needed a stent or stents. That thought did not fill me with delight. Just as I hadn't wanted hip replacements years ago, I wasn't keen on the idea of bits of plastic and metal in my coronary arteries. But God knew best; I had no doubt about that.

I remembered a vision that I had seen in November 2021 and was greatly encouraged. Healing on the Streets had been started in Ballymena in late 2016, and I joined the team from the beginning because of God's call to "carry My healing to others." We had been off the streets during lockdown and were all meeting with the founder of the ministry before re-launching. At the end of the meeting, this gentleman was praying a blessing over the team. Literally simultaneously, just as he said, "God loves your heart," I saw my little physical heart in God's enormous hand and immediately knew that my heart was safe in His care.

Fast forward to July 2022. I had received my appointment to have a CT angiogram with possible stenting in the Royal Victoria Hospital on July 21. I had let my praying friends know and they were praying that all would go well. My prayer was that the narrowing would have opened up and I would not need any stents. One Saturday, I was on the Healing on the Streets team, and my friends wanted to pray for me. I felt a warm tingle go through all of my body as one person in particular prayed, and I was certain that God had touched me.

The following day was Sunday, and my daughter and family had set off early in the morning on holiday, leaving me to look after their cats. I went to the house after the morning church service, and one cat could not be found! How was I going to tell my grandchildren that their cat had disappeared? The other was mewing mournfully for her friend. I searched and searched with no success, and I was distraught.

Over the summer, my church had no evening service so I started going to a small Pentecostal church in a village a few miles from Ballymena on Sunday evenings. As I drove down that road, I started to pray that God would find the missing cat for me and planned to return to the house after church. We had wonderful worship, and then the pastor came to the pulpit. His subject was to be prayer based on John 14:13 *"And whatever you ask in My name, that I will do, that the Father will be glorified in the Son."* The pastor read the Scripture, and then there was a long pause while he was obviously hearing something from God. Then he began, "You could be praying for anything tonight, maybe your cat..." I was astounded.

He went on to preach the wonderful message he had planned, and God spoke to me to remind me that if I could trust Him to find a lost cat, I could trust Him to look after my heart. At the end of the service, I told the pastor that I had been praying for a cat all the way to church and how God had spoken to me. He was glad to know why his sermon didn't start the way he had planned! So what about the cat? I drove to my daughter's house, and there she was waiting at the front door. . Doesn't God speak in amazing ways? Of course I could trust Him with my heart!

The following Sunday was July 17, four days before the procedure. I was truly believing that God had healed me but had decided to keep the appointment in order to testify to the hospital staff. On that Sunday morning, we were singing a modern worship song which says "There is Another in the fire standing next to me, there is Another in the water holding back the sea." Jesus was going to be with me throughout the procedure. The power of God hit me; my knees buckled, and all I remember is trembling uncontrollably on the church floor. I believe a spirit of infirmity left me at that moment, and my healing was complete.

Now you are predicting how this chapter ends too. There's a certain sameness to all these healings. You are absolutely correct if you're assuming I didn't need a stent. Praise God, the previously narrowed area was normal, so nothing needed to be done. I wasn't a great witness due to the administration of strong analgesia, but I did say "Praise the Lord" to the doctor.

However, the procedure was not without complications, but do not let this discourage you if you need to have an angiogram. I am something of a peculiarity! When the cannula was put into the radial artery at my right wrist, the artery went into a spasm, and my forearm became discoloured as well as very painful—so painful that it triggered chest pain and I was given diamorphine which relieved all pain but made me feel very groggy indeed. That is why I was unable to witness as enthusiastically as I had hoped. The doctor was able to proceed as my arteries relaxed, and he gave me the good news that I did not need any stents but had coronary arteries too that were prone to developing spasms. During all this, I developed a bad migraine with flashing lights, a disorientated feeling, and a headache despite the diamorphine. As I would take a migraine occasionally, I was not at all concerned. My Jesus was most definitely with me.

The cardiac specialist recommended starting me on two new drugs to prevent spasms in my arteries. I am deliberately not naming any medication so as not to cause any concern among those who need the drugs and can take them. I would have left out this part of my story, but I wanted to give God the glory for a normal brain scan. I had strange symptoms when I came home from hospital. I was dizzy and unsteady, and I was having some problems finding the correct words when speaking or even texting on my phone. My GP was concerned that I might have had a slight stroke when I thought I was having a migraine, so I was referred very urgently for a brain scan and assessment by a neurologist. My brain scan showed absolutely no abnormality, not even scarring from the healing of multiple sclerosis in 2013, praise God.

The only problem was that the new tablets had lowered my blood pressure far too much. My blood pressure had always been just normal, and the cardiologist had no way of anticipating the effect the medication would have. It took some time for the medication to wear off, but after a couple of weeks I was back to feeling reasonably well and with no chest pains. I will look after my health as best I can and trust God to look after my heart as He has promised.

Chapter 5

Why me?

A few people have asked me that question, and there is no short answer to it. I sometimes even ask God why He has chosen to heal me so many times, and the only thing I know is that God knows I will always testify to His healing power, His love, and His goodness.

I remember some years ago wanting to pray for someone dear to me who was elderly and having joint pains. God told me to ask her what difference it would make to her life if she were healed. I expected her to talk about going for walks and working in the garden—in other words, doing things she previously enjoyed. But God knew what I did not. I'm glad I obeyed and asked the question exactly as He told me to. So, what difference would it make? The answer shocked me. "It would make no difference because I couldn't tell people about it the way you do."

So maybe one reason for my healings is that, although I am by nature a shy person, I am never reluctant to testify to all that God has done for me or to teach, preach, or heal the sick in Jesus' name.

I said at the beginning of the book that this is the story of my journey with Jesus to divine healing. You will have read that each healing came in a different way. Many of them required obedience—doing exactly what God told me to do. All required faith and trust. I believe worship plays a part as well, not only in the shoulder healing. Just as we are to pray without ceasing, I am inclined to worship without ceasing, even if it's just in my mind.

The book is about my Lord, not me. It is about what He has done for me and is willing to do for you too if you go on that journey with Him. You may have to metaphorically push through the crowd to touch the hem of His garment, whatever that may look like in your life.[7] We are all unique, yet made in God's image. Sickness and disease are not God's plan for us, whom He loves.

Believers can all recite John 3:16. Think about God SO loving you that he did not want you to perish but to have eternal life. The sacrifice the Lord Jesus made at Calvary was not only for our salvation but for our healing here on earth as well. When you read through the gospels, did Jesus ever refuse to heal anyone who asked? And note how often healing came in conjunction with forgiveness, which offended the religious people of the day. Is there a lesson there? You probably know about the paralysed man in Capernaum who was let down through the roof of a house by his friends to meet with Jesus. *"But immediately, when Jesus perceived in His spirit that they reasoned thus within themselves, He said to them, "Why do you reason about these things in your hearts? Which is easier, to say to the paralytic, 'Your sins are forgiven you,' or to say, 'Arise, take up your bed and walk'? But that you may know that the Son of Man has power on earth to forgive sins,"* *He said to the paralytic, "I say to you, arise, take up your bed, and go to your house." Immediately he arose, took up the bed, and went out in the presence of them all, so that all were amazed and glorified God, saying, "We never saw anything like this!"* Mark 2:8-12.

"But He was wounded for our transgressions, He was bruised for our iniquities; The chastisement for our peace was upon Him, And by His stripes we are healed." Isaiah 53:5.

---

[7] Matthew 9:20-22.

By His stripes, I am most certainly healed from the following:

- ○ Ankylosing spondylitis and seronegative arthropathy

- ○ Multiple sclerosis

- ○ Irritable bowel syndrome

- ○ Malaria

- ○ A ruptured supraspinatus tendon

- ○ Angina

Do I feel even slightly worthy of such kindness and mercy? Most definitely not. I have failed my Lord so many times in the almost 50 years that I have walked with Him. But every time I fail, He wipes the slate clean and lets me start again. So, while there is breath in my body, I will testify to my salvation, my healings, and the indescribable joy and privilege of being allowed to serve Him in whatever way He calls me to. And I'm very glad that some of that service is in Kenya.

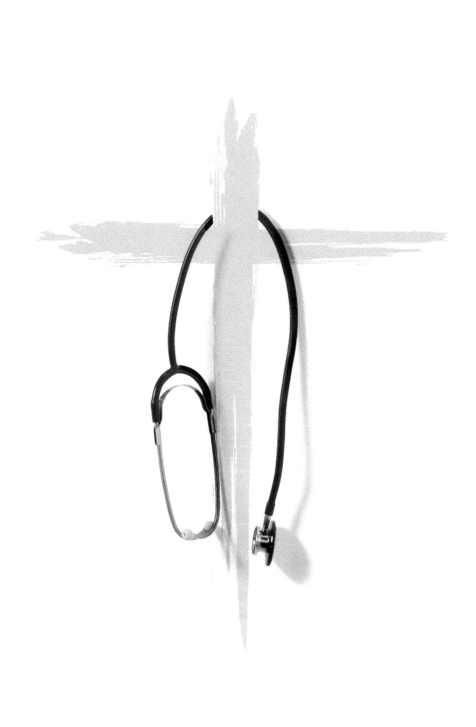

Chapter 6

What if healing does not come?

My initial answer to that question is to persevere in prayer, most certainly. Do not give up. I could probably write another book on blockages to healing. Maybe someday I will. For now, I suggest just a few points.

Do you feel unworthy and undeserving? Then study your identity in Christ. Learn who God says you are.

Is there unconfessed sin in your life? God knows about it anyway. Do not imagine that if you don't talk to God about a sin, He won't find out. He knew before you even committed it. You just have to repent, which is not always easy. But consider the alternative.

Are you holding a grudge or unforgiveness against someone? *"Forgive us our trespasses as we forgive those who trespass against us."* Would you like God to only forgive you to the extent that you forgive some enemy? I shouldn't think so! Unforgiveness is one of the most common causes of physical and mental illness.

Will you lose out financially if disability benefits are stopped? I know that is an issue. I was on disability living allowance when I had ankylosing spondylitis, and we did miss that extra money coming into the home when I was healed. However, being well is definitely preferable.

Does the "sick role" suit you by absolving you of some responsibilities? I don't intend that to sound like a cruel question. It's just something I have seen. For some people, an illness is their easy way out, and they do not truly want to be healed.

Finally, do you want to die? A few years ago, an elderly Christian lady I knew had cancer that had spread all through her body. God showed me clear pictures of all the multiple tumours in that lady's body, so I knew that meant He was willing to heal. He also gave me a word for the lady:

"I don't need the enemy's help to take My children home."

It is understandable in late old age to want to go home to heaven. The mistake people make is thinking that they have to die of an illness. That is not so, which is why God gave me that word for the lady. She did not accept healing and went to be with Jesus a week or so later. The alternative was that her last days would have been perfectly comfortable, and she would still have gone when Jesus called. All sickness is from the enemy, and God has no use for it.

Chapter 7

Keeping one's healing

The enemy's only desire is to steal, kill, and destroy. How he would love to steal my healing, but he cannot unless I make a foolish decision to allow him to do so.

After the healing of my back and joint condition in 2012, I absolutely knew that I was completely and permanently healed. However, a slight muscular pain which we all experience from time to time, would cause the enemy to whisper "You're not really healed." I could only reply, like Jesus during His temptation in the wilderness, with *"It is written..."* God promised *"I am the Lord that heals you"*, Exodus 15:26. I could list many more Scriptures promising healing—here are just a few:

"Let all that I am praise the Lord; may I never forget the good things he does for me. He forgives all my sins and heals all my diseases." Psalm 103:2-3

"I will give you back your health and heal your wounds," says the Lord." Jeremiah 30:17

I know that I have to keep actively believing that my healings are permanent. Everything in God's Word implies that they are. And I believe my healings are all complete; throughout the gospels when Jesus healed anyone, He healed completely, and there is no record of anyone's sickness returning.

I know that the words I speak about myself are crucially important. *"Death and life are in the power of the tongue,"* Proverbs 18:21. Therefore, I take ownership of no diagnosis. I never spoke of "my angina." My blood sugars are a little high but there is no "my diabetes." There is a metabolic upset which God will heal. I have a tendency to mild asthma since childhood, but I never speak of "my asthma." I do not accept it; it is not welcome in my body and some day it will be gone in Jesus' name.

Sadly, many people curse themselves. "I'll never be well." "I've always had poor health." "This condition runs in my family, so I can't avoid it." "Doctors can do no more for me. It's terminal."

All such statements open the door for the enemy to come into agreement with whoever makes them and ensure faithless predictions become reality, sadly.

So, another important factor in maintaining your healing is speaking God's truth about yourself regularly, not only to yourself but also sharing your testimony with others. I am tremendously blessed every time I testify in public to all that God has done in my life.

My final advice is to live worthy of your calling (Ephesians 4:1). If you had to repent of any sin before receiving your healing, be especially careful to never be lured back into such sin again.

If you, like myself, learned many lessons on your journey to healing, do not forget those lessons. Memories can fade with the passage of time. Part of my reason for writing this book is so that I will not forget my precious journeys with my Lord to healing. Write down what you learn, even if no one but yourself will ever read it.

Chapter 8

"Now Carry My Healing to others"

That was quite a calling—a rather daunting one at first, but now a tremendous privilege.

I got no encouragement from my then church leadership initially, but with the benefit of hindsight, I can understand why to a certain extent. I was only in the church a few months when I received my first healing, and God spoke so clearly to me, but it was wisdom for them to wait and see how I turned out.

The person who encouraged me most initially was Wesley Kerr of Life-line Ministries (Ireland), who let me go on a mission trip to Kenya in 2013 and expected all the team to pray for the sick. The first healing that I was aware of was a lady with HIV who testified a few days after I had prayed for her that she knew she had been healed. She is, of course, still alive and well 10 years later. Often in Kenya, because of the language barrier, I don't know what is wrong with the person I'm praying for, but many still testify afterwards to being touched by God. I remember particularly preaching one Saturday in one of our churches when a young mother rushed in carrying a very ill baby. The pastor of the church interrupted the meeting and asked me to pray for the child. The doctor in me was thinking hospital, intravenous fluids, antibiotics—but this was Kenya. All I could do was pray. The next day, being Sunday, the little baby was toddling around his thankful parents in church! Praise God. Did he have malaria or septicaemia? I don't know, but knowing the One who does know is always enough.

I remember once being on a mission trip to Ethiopia, and a young man in the team developed severe upper abdominal pain going through to his back as well as vomiting up blood and passing black bowel motions. I knew this was at least a bleeding duodenal ulcer or maybe even a perforated ulcer. He was in agonising pain, pale, and clammy. We had been advised before going that hospital care was not an option if anyone took ill. So we needed a miracle. I laid hands on him and prayed and prayed. If I stopped praying for a moment, he begged me to pray more. Eventually, after I don't know how long, peace came. I believe he was slain in the spirit for a little while and then was able to tell me that the pain had gone and there was no further blood loss. God was our only hope in that place, and He never fails.

I was once asked to go to pray for a man who was critically ill with septicaemia in the ICU of a hospital in Northern Ireland. This was before Covid, so I was allowed to go in to pray, but the nurse explained that his condition was so critical that she could not leave the room. The man and his fiancée were not believers, and I was their last resort. He was on full life support (ventilator, dialysis, etc.) as all his organs were failing. I placed my hand on his forehead, which was cold and waxy, and for a split second, my flesh told me I was too late, but then faith took over and I prayed my best prayer, commanding all infection to depart in the name of Jesus and all organs to be refreshed and restored back to the way God created them to be. Once I felt I had done all I could, I left. About ten minutes later, I received a text on my phone to say that the nurse had remarked that the patient's blood pressure had started to improve when I was praying and was continuing to improve, having previously been extremely low. By the next day, the patient was becoming aware, and the day after that, he was off the ventilator and had progressed to make a full recovery. Sadly, because he was unconscious, he doesn't really know what an amazing miracle happened. But his partner knows, and the nurse knows. The Holy Spirit can do the rest.

You will notice I am being deliberately vague about who people are because these are their stories to tell, if they would only tell them.

I have the privilege of praying for many people through Healing on the Streets. This ministry is in many towns across the United Kingdom and in other countries too. As all such ministries should be, everything people confide in us is and will remain completely confidential.

During lockdown, I became involved with the Global Prophetic Alliance's Miracle Clinic over Zoom, but my personal preference is for hands-on ministry. *"They will lay hands on the sick and they will recover,"* Mark 16:18. When God told me to Carry His Healing to others, I understood the word "carry" to involve using my hands, and God has never told me otherwise. However, I am very willing to speak forth a healing word in faith to anyone I cannot meet in person.

Just as Jesus never turned anyone away who wanted to be healed, I hope and trust that I never will either. It is my privilege to pray with anyone and minister healing as Jesus told the disciples to and intends all believers to still obey today.

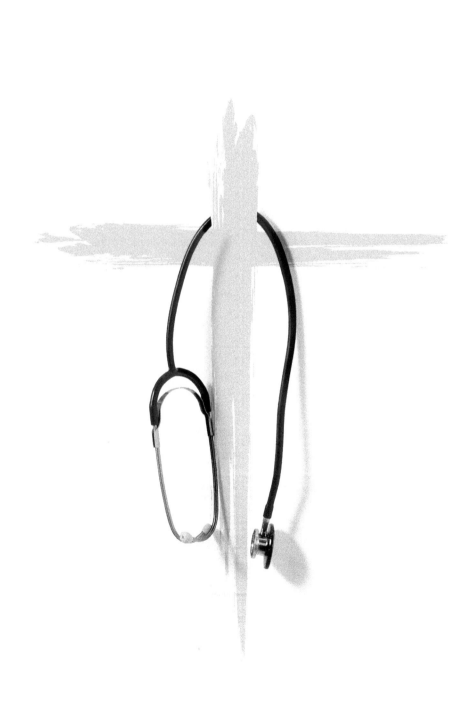

Chapter 9

After Covid, 2022

The travel restrictions during Covid had been especially hard for me, as I was in the habit of going on a mission trip to Kenya at least once a year. When the restrictions were lifted, naturally, the founder of the ministry went first, and then I was advised to wait until after the elections in August 2022. Finally, praise God, I was able to set off on September 21. As always, the plan was that I would visit several Life-line Ministries churches, teach up to three seminars some days, and pray individually with church members. I had not preached in a church for 3 years due to Covid, so I was perhaps a little apprehensive. I needn't have been. I was forgetting God's promise from the previous year; *"When I have tested you, you shall come forth as gold."*[8] As I began to preach and teach, I was hearing a different Audrey, and the pastors realised that too. My suffering with my shoulder had not been in vain. God had done something new in me—something different and precious. I had no concern for what anyone thought of me. I spoke out whatever words God gave me, obediently. All that mattered to me was preaching the Word of God and leading people to Jesus, as well as teaching and encouraging the believers. There was a new fire in me, and I was so thankful to God. Many in the churches knew of my earlier healings, and what a joy to tell them about the enemy's attempt to restrict my worship and how gloriously God healed me again.

Some of my time was spent with the street children in the town of Kitale. I had become aware of their plight during my first trip to

[8] Job 23:10.

Kenya in 2013. We didn't often have reason to be in the town as our churches are in rural villages, but for some reason we were there one day and had gone into a cafe for some lunch. When we came out, a little boy was standing with cupped hands and pleading eyes, begging for us to give him something. At that time, I had two grandsons, aged five and nine. This boy looked between their ages, roughly seven. He was homeless and begging on the streets for food. My heart broke in that moment, and that was the beginning of years of prayer for that little boy and other street children. I still remember that little face so clearly and have not been able to find him since. I do hope he found a home somewhere, but being realistic, that may not be so. Only God knows.

I was thankful when I heard from one of our church members a couple of years ago that he was befriending the street children and initially, just once a month, was able to give them a proper meal. Life-line Ministries became involved, and the children now receive a meal twice a week as well as hearing the Word of God. It was my privilege to join with the volunteers three times and preach the gospel to around one hundred homeless children and teenagers. I was so blessed to see so many respond and accept Jesus as Lord and Saviour. Obviously, they now need to be discipled as most are not from Christian backgrounds and many are illiterate, so they could not read Bibles even if we provided them.

While in the Kitale area, I was taken to see a house that was available for rent, and some of our church members felt it would be an ideal home for the youngest street children. I agreed wholeheartedly, and with donated money, was able to pay rent in advance and arrange for the purchase of basic essentials such as mattresses, blankets and kitchen equipment. At the time of writing, I am trusting God for regular provision to keep the home running. The streets are not safe for anyone to live on, but especially not for young children, who are in danger from older boys and anyone abusing alcohol, etc. So, I know God's blessing will rest on all we do to help these children.

While I was still in Kenya but had moved on to Kisumu, we got the sad news that a young street boy in Kitale had been assaulted by an older boy and died of his injuries. That further added to my determination to rescue the youngest and most vulnerable children and give them a safe home where they will be well cared for and be brought up in a Christian environment, as well as being able to go to a local primary school and Life-line church.

I really cherished the opportunities to teach the Word of God in our Life-line churches. Each week I was there, I taught three seminars on Friday and Saturday and then spoke at the Sunday service. It never ceases to amaze me that pastors are eager for me to teach in their churches and are themselves blessed as I do so. That can only be God! As I remind the church members, I am nobody special in the natural. I'm just an ordinary wife, mother, and grandmother—just an ordinary woman who passionately loves Jesus. Surely the Lord is willing to use anyone who is willing to allow Him to.

May you be encouraged to keep seeking God for any healing you need and to pursue His perfect will for your life. You will never regret doing so, that's for certain!

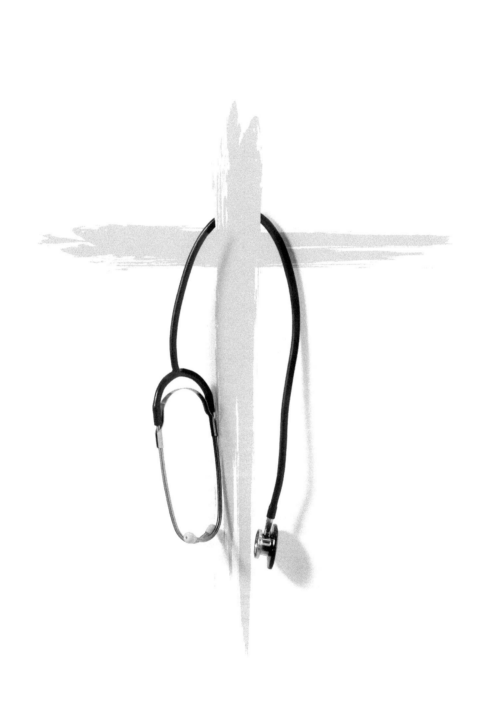

Chapter 10

April 2023

Over the winter months, much had been happening in Kenya. Wesley Kerr, the founder of Life-line ministries, spent some time there and was able to help with the practical work involved in making the building I had seen in September 2022 fully ready to become our children's home. Eight children, three boys and five girls, were selected from the street children who attended the feeding programme regularly. They were aged from three and a half up to eleven. Imagine a little girl of three living on the streets or in a dump and scavenging for food! You will understand that my heart is frequently broken. But imagine, if we can try, how our Father God feels! One other little boy has now come under our care since I returned home, so we now have nine precious children in total.

I had been asked to return to Kenya once the children had time to settle in, to get to know them as little individuals. But God had other plans too. Certainly, time was spent with the children. They were bought extra clothes, including school uniforms, to take the pressure off the carers concerning washing. They also received extra blankets, as despite their life on the streets, some were finding their bunks cold. They also got casual track suits and clothes for church on Sundays. Some storage cupboards and shelves were needed, as were a dining table and two sofas. So, the home is definitely more homely-looking now than when I arrived, but the children all knew before this that they were very much loved. I will never forget them singing "We welcome you, Mummy, we love you, Mummy." Only someone with a heart of stone would not be touched. However, that does not alter the fact that children's ministry has never been my calling; it is not now, and I have no reason to think it ever will be. Praise God, I am not needed to teach these children the Word of God. They attend Sunday school and church, and their carers are committed Christian women from our own local Life-line church. These women and Sunday school teachers have a calling and an anointing that I do not have. My callings are healing ministry, evangelism, and teaching believers, but I care about children just as many other mothers and grandmothers do—on a natural level. It may be that losing my father at the age of eleven and knowing that my dear mother faced many struggles, has made me that bit more sensitive to the needs of orphaned or abandoned children, and that could be part of God's plan. Over nearly fifty years with my Lord, I have learned to hear His voice so clearly, and my only agenda is to obey His call.

Supernaturally strange things were happening on this mission trip. God had instilled greater boldness in me to teach on such topics as the reverential fear of God, which is missing in so many churches worldwide. The next topic was the abuse of grace. I had preached in fellowship meetings on true freedom in Christ. These were not lessons for little children! Again, God was reminding me that children's ministry wasn't my calling, and I was not to be distracted from my true purpose.

The last day of my trip was spent at a youth conference in Eldoret, where I had been invited to be the guest speaker. I am very happy to teach teens and twenties, maybe because it is part of Kenyan culture to show respect for the older generation; therefore, I don't have to fear having anything thrown at me! The theme of the conference was revival, and I attempted to address some of the possible reasons why we no longer see the wonderful revivals of centuries past. I encouraged the young people that revival begins in each of us and that we are called individually to lives of holiness (*"Be holy as I am holy,"* 1 Peter 1:16) and that God will only use clean vessels (*"that each of you should know how to possess his own vessel in sanctification and honour,"* 1 Thessalonians 4:4). I encouraged these precious young people to study and obey God's Word with the help of the Holy Spirit and to pray that revival will come again.

All too soon, it was time to start the homeward journey from Eldoret to Nairobi, then on to Istanbul, and finally to Dublin. For some reason of which we were never advised, the flight from Nairobi was delayed by over two hours. I began to realise that unless my next flight was also delayed, I would also miss it and be stranded in Istanbul. This was a Saturday morning, and I had been in airports or on planes from 6 pm on Friday. I was utterly exhausted. Time to start declaring the word of God and in the circumstances, my chosen scripture was Romans 8:28, *"All things work together for good to those who love God, to those who are the called according to His purposes."* I love God, and I am called by God, so I could believe all things would work together for my good. Did we avoid a plane crash by being late? Only God knows.

I was waiting, rather wearily admittedly, in Istanbul to hear when I could get to Dublin. When told it would not be until Sunday morning, I imagined trying to rest on the airport floor, and a tear almost escaped. I just wanted to be home with my husband and family by this stage. But then there was a surprise. I was to be taken by minibus to a hotel and brought back to the airport on time for my flight. What sort of hotel would it be? Please, Lord, no bed bugs! I had met them in 2016, and that was enough.

I need not have doubted. My hotel was five-star and part of a well-known European chain. It was comfortable in every way, and every need was provided for. I would have been happy in a simple bed and breakfast, but here I was in a luxury hotel! I was indeed seeing all things working together for good and had several hours of sound sleep before it was time to return to Istanbul airport.

That morning, the flight took off on time and arrived in Dublin after 10 a.m. Now I just had to get my luggage and find a bus going to Belfast. If only! I waited and waited, but my suitcase did not come along the carousel. The other passengers drifted off one by one, and there I stood, with no luggage, literally just holding my handbag, and wearing a summer dress and a cardigan at the end of April. All my warmer clothes were in that missing suitcase, along with my precious old, tattered study Bible. That was the beginning of filling out an online report and other paperwork. I heard some passengers being told their luggage would be delivered the following day. When I inquired it seemed my luggage had not left Nairobi! I was told I could only wait while the airline did their best to try to find my missing baggage. So I went home and slept and slept. Monday came and passed with more sleep but no news. Hope was waning. Maybe I should submit a claim to my travel insurance. Then on Tuesday night, there was a knock at the front door, and I was reunited with my dirty washing but, most importantly, with my old study bible and various other books.

I realise that the missed connection was maybe God's way of telling me that splitting a long journey would be a good idea as I get older. And was the delayed luggage to make me rest before starting unpacking and washing? Only God knows, but I do know this: my God is interested in every aspect of my life, however trivial, even missed flights and delayed baggage. But He is interested in so much more! He knows every fleeting thought before I've started to think about it; He knows every slightest concern I might have about myself or a loved one; He knows the answer to every question before it has formed in my mind. My Creator, God, knows everything about me. I can have no secrets from Him. No matter what my circumstances, God is Sovereign, and He will take control if I ask Him to.

I am surrounded by sad, confused, anxious and distraught people seeking guidance and a purpose in life who do not have to live that way. God is waiting for someone reading this to cry out to Him and to hear Him reply as He did to me:

"You do not have because you do not ask," James 4:2.

"So I say to you, ask and it will be given to you, seek and you will find," Luke 11:9.

Chapter 11

It is not over for you!

I hope, if you have read this far, that God has spoken to you according to your needs. God knew everything about me: every foolish thought, every false belief, every correct and sincere belief, and every good intention. One of the many blessings of reaching late middle age (I'm not elderly yet!) is that there are many years to think back over. As I think back over the decades, God was always at work in my life. In my earlier years, I couldn't always see it. Now I do. I often ask God to show me how He wants to use me today, and I try very hard to listen and obey. Do I ever miss what God has for me now? I have no doubt that I do, because I will not be perfect until God takes me home.

I hope the story of my journey with Jesus will encourage new believers and those young in the faith to persevere. Look how many years I suffered needlessly, but I had to be in the right place in my deepening relationship with the Lord before I could receive my healing. I have no doubt that healing is always God's will, but sometimes people will not fully surrender to receive His will. How my heart aches when I pray for someone's healing, and I sense that resistance in their spirit. How it must grieve the Lord Jesus Christ, who suffered so greatly at the whipping post and on the cross so that we can be healed, and people reject His offer? Why will people gladly receive salvation but ignore the fact that Jesus suffered and died for their healing as well as for their salvation? I leave the reader with that question to ponder.

I do understand that, having been a doctor for many years, readers may wonder how I feel about medical treatments now. I do believe that God can use medical or surgical treatments to heal if He so chooses, and I would never discourage anyone from seeking medical advice or treatment. I wish to make that clear. To do less would be irresponsible.

However, this book is about my *personal* experience of medical treatments and divine healing. All the medication for ankylosing spondylitis left me with slightly impaired kidney function, which, praise God, has not worsened since stopping the treatment. I think it is reasonable to say that it did not benefit me in any way.

I received no treatment for multiple sclerosis, irritable bowel syndrome, malaria, or the shoulder injury, and I know it was God who healed each condition.

I agreed to take a statin to lower the cholesterol level in my blood in the hope of reducing the likelihood of other coronary artery blockages, as well as aspirin to make my blood less sticky. I do not for a moment think that the statin removed the obstruction in my left anterior descending coronary artery. I give God the glory for that, in addition to all my other healings. The cardiologists say I have arteries which are prone to go into spasms, but I was unable to tolerate their recommended medication, so I trust God to look after every part of my heart as I know He has promised to do. It is only common sense to keep to as healthy a lifestyle as I can manage, and I have no objection to taking drugs such as statins or aspirin, which work in conjunction with a healthy diet and exercise, while they cause no side effects. What I can say for certain is that the angina I used to experience has not recurred since the experience I described, when I believe a spirit of infirmity left my body.

The wonderful thing about a testimony is that nobody can argue with it. I experienced what I've experienced, and no medical professional can say I didn't, no matter how bizarre they may think my story is. When I was eventually seen at an NHS orthopaedic clinic regarding my shoulder, the clinician could not understand how I was pain-free and had full shoulder movements despite what the ultrasound and MRI scans showed. Sadly, she could not accept that I had been healed by God but agreed that nobody can deny my experience. I wasn't offered a repeat scan, and I would not have accepted it anyway, as it would have been a waste of resources and would change nothing. God restored my shoulder to a normally functioning and pain-free shoulder in the way He chose, and He did so suddenly at the moment of His choosing.

I hope you have enjoyed and been blessed by reading about my journey through healings. I tell my story mainly to glorify God and to praise Him for all He has done in my life, but also to encourage anyone battling with health problems. Please believe that God wants to heal you as He healed me. Start off on your personal journey with Jesus to divine healing. Whatever health problems you are struggling with, God knows all about them, and your story is not over yet. I urge you to seek Him, wait on Him, and listen to Him while believing that your healing is His will.

May my story give hope and encouragement wherever it is needed, in Jesus' name.

To learn more about Dr Audrey Johnston's ministry,
obtain free teachings and purchase books, visit:

www.CarryMyHealing.com

INSPIRED TO WRITE A BOOK?

Contact

Maurice Wylie Media

Your Inspirational & Christian Book Publisher

Based in Northern Ireland and distributing around the world.

www.MauriceWylieMedia.com

.

Milton Keynes UK
Ingram Content Group UK Ltd.
UKHW021018181023
430759UK00010B/62